In Fond Memory

Catherine M Bowlby
a creative inspiration

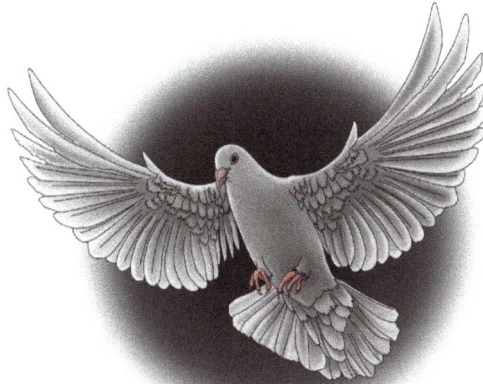

SOLDIERS STORIES UNWOUND

Aromatherapy for Veterans with PTSD

Elaine Bowlby, LAc.

First published in the United States in 2021

Book Design and Graphics by Carla Millar

Point Location diagrams by Acudude.

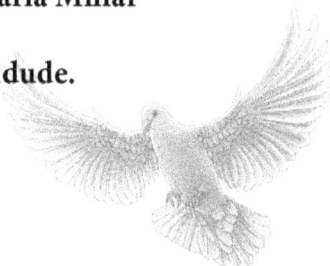

ISBN: 9780578949789

Note: An Asterix * indicates a reference to the Healing Oil Collective by Tiffany Pollard, LAc, MH
Caution: The information given in this book is not intended to be a substitute for medical treatment or diagnosis. Organic Essential Oils are powerful and are to be used in appropriate dilutions with appropriate age groups. Qualified practitioners should be consulted in the aromatherapy field if there is a doubt or question about their usage.

Contents

Foreword

This was a labor of love, love, love. Although I have never served my country in a military capacity, I am part of a military family, which has given me some insights into the issues of soldiers. My intentions are two fold, to give practitioners another tool to address the needs of their veteran patients, as well as to serve these very same warriors, who have consistently put their lives on the line. Inspiration was sourced from the life of St Ignasius, a dedicated soldier who turned to spiritual life after being wounded during battle. This birthed a comprehensive guide of inspired elixirs and essential oil protocols that comprise Soldiers Stories Unwound. The collection is designed to treat trauma conditions characteristically experienced by veterans; such as ADD, PTSD and insomnia, plus emotional states such as guilt, anguish and anger. The following pages include the ingredients and practical applications of the collection, as well as, point location diagrams, home remedies and the effects of each oil or essence. This guide draws on my education and experience in Acupuncture, Chinese herbal medicine and Aromatherapy over the last 20 years. This includes the application of essential oils on acupuncture points, called Aroma Point Therapy or Aroma Acupoint Therapy. In this technique, the essential oil enhances the functions of the points and vice versa. This allows for healing on a number of levels.

I would like to acknowledge my teachers of this extraordinary technique and therapy, Peter Holmes, LAc, MH and Tiffany Pollard, LAc, MH. They literally opened up a whole new world to me, filled with the science of plant essences and their wondrous healing properties. I often refer to their teachings in this guide and my words can never fully express my gratitude.

The protocols outlined here are designed to be used in conjunction with the elixirs that make up the Soldiers Stories Unwound collection found at www.soulswaywellness.com. The elixirs are blended for adults 18 years of age and above. Precautions are required for use with pregnant women and those on medications or with skin sensitivities. Be advised that one elixir contains trace amounts of alcohol as a preservative, and should be used with caution on patients with addictions to alcoholic substances. Questions or comments are welcome and can be directed to the author at soulswaywellness@gmail.com.

"Forgiveness"

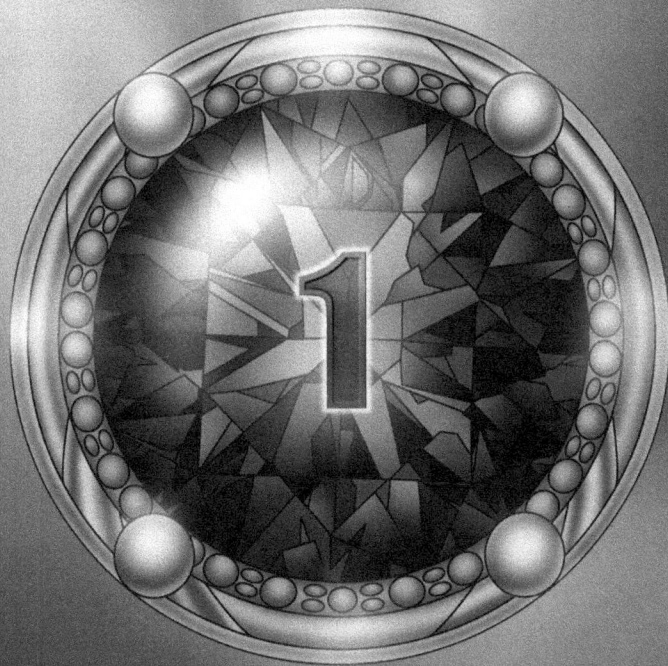

SOLDIERS STORIES UNWOUND

"Forgiveness"

The first of the five protocols that comprises Soldiers Stories Unwound is Forgiveness. This essential oil blend is important for combat soldiers who have taken the life of another or who were witness to this loss of life. The intention of the soldier is paramount to the usage of this blend, i.e., the protection of homeland and/or ideals of freedom, preservation of future generations, etc... This blend will not be effective in other circumstances of life loss, including friendly fire, accidents or cases of murder. This protocol has a component integral in freeing dead souls that have become attached to the surviving soldier's energetic field during combat. As the soul(s) detach and find their true home, there is a self forgiveness that needs to happen before any other symptoms can be addressed. Transformational healing is only made possible through forgiveness of self, as well as forgiveness of others. The star in this pursuit is rose, hence the use of damask rose in the protocol itself, as well as in the compounding process through diffusion and the use of the rose quartz crystal.

Forgiveness Elixir In Jojoba Carrier Oil

Ingredients: Black Spruce, Frankincense, Damask Rose, Blue Tansy, Marjoram, Cardamon, Ravintsara, Juniper Berry, Atlas Cedarwood, Vetiver, Saro, and Ylang Ylang Essential Oils.
Elixir is blended on the Flower of Life grid with Rose Quartz while diffusing Damask Rose Essential Oil, calling upon Arch Angel Michael's protection.

"Forgiveness"

Aroma Acupoint Protocol

The direct contact, galaxy cotton ball or double tipped cotton stick method can be used in this protocol. See pages 52-53 for descriptions of suggested application methods. The direct contact method is described in protocol below. Start treatment with patient lying in a supine position.

1. ST41 - put 1-2 drops of Forgiveness Elixir on one index finger and transfer to second index finger by pressing fingers lightly together. Place both index fingers on ST41 bilaterally. Hold lightly for 60 plus seconds until a shift occurs.
2. CV6 - put 1-2 drops of Forgiveness Elixir on index finger. Hold lightly for 60 plus seconds until shift occurs. Entire palm of hand can be placed over point as well, while waiting for a shift.
3. GV11 - After applying 1-2 drops of Elixir to index or middle finger, slide hand between patient and treatment table and hold on point until shift occurs. Holding flat palms on CV6 and GV11 simultaneously for a few more seconds can be comforting to patient, depending on the individual. Alternately, you may flip the patient to a prone position before applying the Elixir to GV11. In this case, I suggest treating GV11 solely, waiting for 60 plus seconds and/or shift in energy.

"Forgiveness"

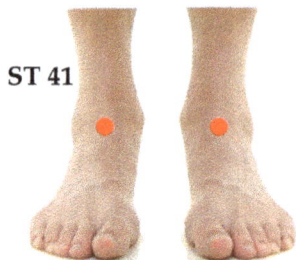

ST 41

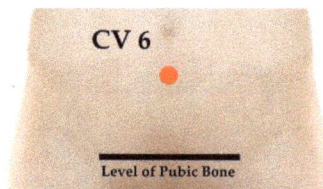

CV 6

Level of Pubic Bone

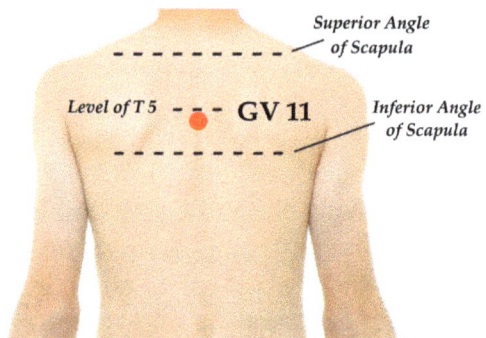

Superior Angle of Scapula

Level of T 5 **GV 11**

Inferior Angle of Scapula

"Forgiveness"

Point Location and Functions

ST41 - Jiexi/Ravine Divide - At the midpoint of the transverse crease of the ankle, level with the tip of the external malleolus, in the depression between the tendons of extensor digitorum longus and hallucis longus.

Addresses opposite end channel issues, i.e., restless leg syndrome and mania; clears the brain and is used to treat ADD and ADHD.

CV6 - Qi Hai/Sea of Qi - Midway between CV5 and CV7, 1.5 cun below the umbilicus (CV8).

Generally useful for Qi tonification. Gathers scattered Qi and brings one back to authentic self.

GV11 - Shen Dao/Spirit Path - Under the spinous process of T5 at the midline of the spine, located behind the heart.

Shen Dao is an important point for problems with spirit, palpitations, anxiety, poor memory, muddled thinking and absent mindedness. It addresses insomnia and has a strong effect on mind and mood.

"Forgiveness"

Essences and Their Functions

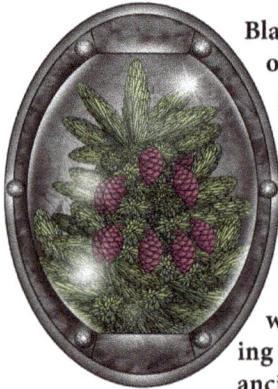

Black Spruce (*Picea mariana*) is a revered essential oil, not only because of it's range of therapeutic effects, but also because it connects us to our prenatal energies. As such, Black Spruce has been called the "Parter of Veils" and the "Bridge between Worlds" by Tiffany Pollard, LAc, MH. These nomenclatures indicate Black Spruce's role in the transition of souls to their rightful home. In addition to this function, this oil is helpful with grief, anxiety, withdrawal, depression and despair at the deepest levels. This essential oil is obtained from the fresh needles and twigs of the conifer tree whose scent is clarifying and invigorating with deep woody, earthy and musky undertones. This oil is also tonifying and supports immunity. Partnered here with Frankincense, both these ancient oils are central to transitioning souls in this essential oil blend.

Black Spruce

Frankincense (*Boswellia carterii*) is The Great Connector* and the Rainbow Bridge* to the other side and is considered one of the most sacred essential oils. It is one of the thick essential oils that is considered closest to Original Source. As such, Frankincense is used in this elixir to aid Black Spruce in returning detached souls back to Source. This essential oil is distilled from the resin of the Boswellia tree of Somalia. The resin is obtained by slashing the bark of the tree. The resultant thick, milky substance is the tree's attempt to heal itself. This response reflects the ability of Frankincense to treat both physical and emotional wounds that have not yet healed. It increases the depth of respiration, allows for forgiveness and taking in new life while letting go of the past. Frankincense eases grief and can bring clarity to life situations.

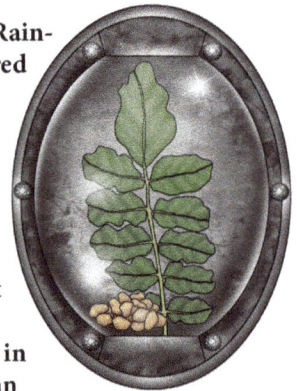

Frankincense

6

"Forgiveness"

Essences and Their Functions

Damask Rose (*Rosa damascena*) imparts Compassionate Grace*. It is the One* who evokes compassionate acceptance of self and engenders a field of forgiveness. It is the last function of facilitating forgiveness that is most important in this elixir. This includes both forgiveness of self and that of others. Rose's sweet aromatic scent softens the hardened or armored heart and invites it to gently open, allowing the tenderness of forgiveness to enter. Rose essential oil reminds us, that despite our wounds, we are whole and ever new.* Rose can help resolve feelings of shame and anger turned inward, as well as other feelings that contribute to self sabotage. It also helps heal the heart damaged by patterns of domination/ submission and abuse. Because Rose is balancing, calming and nuturing, it can also help with mood swings, low self esteem and feelings of anxiety, depression, jealousy and envy. Rose Essential oil is obtained through steam distillation of organic blossoms of Rosa damascena from Bulgaria.

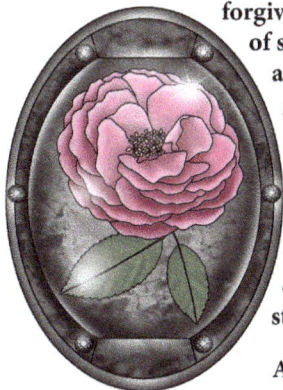

As Damask Rose has an affinity to the heart, Blue Tansy (*Tanacetum annuum*) has to the pericardium and liver. Because the pericardium protects the heart, sometimes it is imperative to treat the pericardium along with the heart, so the desired effects will be realized. Blue Tansy essential oil "lightens the load" as it is the essence of play. Blue Tansy is likened to the Court Jester;* whose truth telling is tolerated because of his/her directness and humor. Therefore, it is calming, soothing and refreshing simultaneously. Blue Tansy relieves stress, tension, anxiety and worry. It also addresses symptoms usually associated with Liver Stagnation in Chinese medicine; feelings of frustration, irritability and oversensitivity. The essential oil is extracted from the fresh Moroccan herb and fresh flowering buds by steam distillation. It's color is a calming marine blue due to it's Chamazulene content. It has an intense sweet green and fruity scent with spicy undertones.

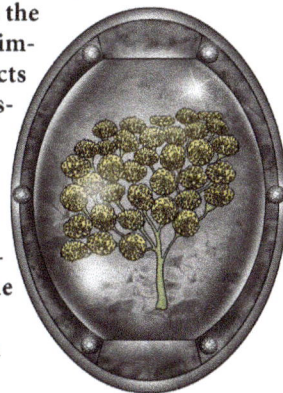

Damask Rose

Blue Tansy

"Forgiveness"

Essences and Their Functions

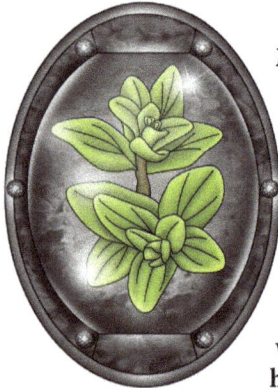

Marjoram (*Origanum maiorana*) is a dual action essential oil as it has both relaxant and restorative properties. This sweet-herbaceous essential oil relaxes the mind/body/spirit. Emotionally, it relaxes automatic resistance to inside/outside stimuli, as it also restores healthy boundaries without undo influence of the past.* Physically, marjoram relaxes the armature of the muscle body, including the heart muscle, facilitating the release of traumatic muscle memories that no longer serve. Marjoram is used in this blend for it's calming, cooling and balancing effects emotionally, while providing relaxing, warming and antispasmodic qualities for the physical body. The human body recognizes this herb as food with it's long history of use in cuisine, which allows the body to be most receptive to it's effects.

Marjoram

Cardamon (*Elettaria cardamomum*) is another herb that has a history of use in our kitchens, reflecting it's nourishing properties to the physical as well as the spiritual body. Warming, uplifting and energizing, cardamon essential oil stimulates mental, physical and emotional functions. This aromatic spicy oil aids poor concentration and memory loss while addressing digestion, tiredness or exhaustion with depression. It has the emotional affect of getting a big, comforting hug. Cardamon essential oil is distilled from cardamon pods from Sri Lanka. It's warm nature helps to circulate and encourage the heart to reconnect, which makes it a great asset to the purpose of this blend.

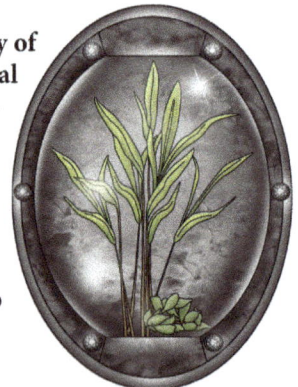

8

Cardamon

"Forgiveness"

Essences and Their Functions

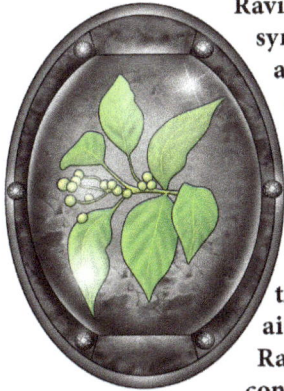

Ravintsara (*Cinnamomum camphora cineole*) is used here to aid with symptoms of ADD and depression, which is common in soldiers in the aftermath of combat. This essential oil is obtained from distillation of the fresh leaves of the camphor tree from Madagascar and has actions that are uplifting, refreshing, warming and drying. Ravintsara strengthens weak conditions, including chronic mental and physical fatigue, low self confidence, and difficulty making decisions. It also exerts a deeply restoring action on nervous, cerebral and immune functions. Therefore, this fresh pungent oil addresses loss of motivation and self esteem, helps with the inability to move forward; as well as aid with problems of insomnia and upper/lower respiratory infections. Ravintsara is contraindicated in cases of pregnancy and should not be confused with Ravensara (*Ravensara aromatic*) which has less therapeutic functions and whose tree is an endangered species.

Ravintsara

Juniper Berry (*Juniperus communis*) is another oil that addresses symptoms of depression, disempowerment, as well as those of self neglect. These symptoms often occur when there is lack of forgiveness, especially forgiveness of self, which makes juniper berry a great addition to this blend. The best quality Juniper Berry oil is a steam distillation of the fresh or dried ripe berries. It's fresh spicy, fruity, green and woody aroma promotes clarity, self confidence, motivation and endurance; helpful in cases of mental disorientation, spaciness, lethargy and discouragement. Juniper Berry is a warming, drying stimulant and can be used in chronic flaccid, cold conditions and chronic rheumatic and arthritic conditions. It is contraindicated in cases of pregnancy, because of it's uterine stimulant action; and kidney disease, because of its diuretic action.

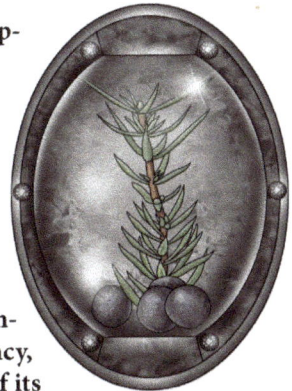

Juniper Berry

"Forgiveness"

Essences and Their Functions

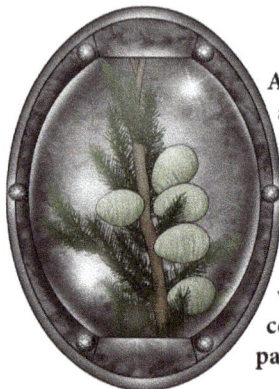

Atlas Cedarwood (*Cedrus atlantica*) essential oil is warming, strengthening, and inviting. This rich, sweet woody oil is obtained through steam distillation of the dried wood shavings from the heartwood of this majestic tree of North Morocco's Atlas Mountains. Atlas Cedarwood conveys a strength and permanency that few trees possess. It is one of the oldest conifers in existence and can live for centuries. The timeless strength and stability this conifer imparts is present in the essential oil it produces. Atlas cedarwood treats conditions that are both weak and tense as the oil is bracing, centering and calming. It can address emotional states from anxiety and paranoia to euphoria and delusion, and is indicated in treating ADHD. Both Atlas Cedarwood and Vetiver are used here for their grounding function. Atlas Cedarwood is warm and grounding while it's counterpart, Vetiver, is cool and grounding; the perfect balance of yin and yang.

Atlas Cedarwood

Vetiver (*Vetiveria zizanioides*) is a viscous dark amber or olive oil with deep earthy, rooty aromas often with different notes; which allows for a number of aromatic variants. The essential oil is obtained by steam distillation of the dried roots and rhizomes of this grass family plant from Madagascar. Vetiver is cool and tranquil which engenders the characteristics of deep, mysterious waters. It's long root system offers sustenance, stability and restorative powers to this oil's therapeutic properties. It's used in chronic weak, tense and hot conditions and as a nervous sedative for emotional states with heat; as anxiety with anger. It's supportive, sensual nature addresses disassociation and disconnection, by bringing one back to the physical body. This attribute makes Vetiver important in cases of shock or trauma. In general, Vetiver is the essence of mother earth, or Gaia, as she imparts the deep connection to all of life through her nourishing, empowering nature.

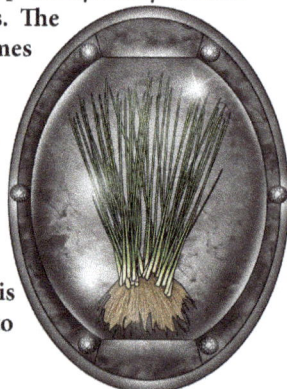

10

Vetiver

"Forgiveness"

Essences and Their Functions

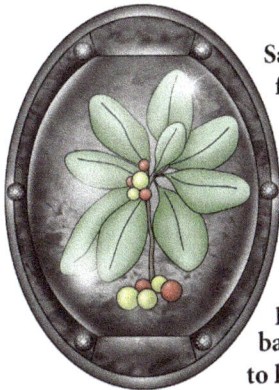

Saro (*Cinnamosma fragrans*) is an understudied but engaging plant from Madagascar. The essential oil is obtained by steam distillation of the fresh leaves. It has a camphoraceous fragrance profile with smooth, warm, sweet and slightly spicy middle notes that is uplifting, vitalizing as well as decongesting. Generally, it is used to support immunity, but in this blend, its primarily used for it's emotional and spiritual properties. Saro opens and reconnects us to ourselves, to others and to universal energies. It imparts a dignified, connected presence. This essential oil encourages a shift from a disconnected ego based power to a true power that is connected to source. It allows one to live from a trusting, integrated space.

Saro

Ylang Ylang (*Cananga odorata*) is translated "flower of flowers" and has a sweet, sensual scent emanating from it's yellow star shaped blossoms. The scent is so deep that the oil is extracted by a fractionated distillation method. Ylang ylang I from Madagascar is the oil extraction used in this blend. It is described as cooling, euphoric, sensual, charismatic and uplifting; characteristics that can be imparted to the user. Ylang ylang is predominantly associated with the Heart and addresses anxiety, tension, palpitations, anger and insomnia, as well as shock or trauma. The essential oil can induce a state of euphoria and optimism that has been described as being in a "protective bubble". This stabilizing effect on moods and emotions is the main reason Ylang ylang is used here. Saro essential oil opens the soul-body to connection and Ylang ylang makes it feel safe to do so.

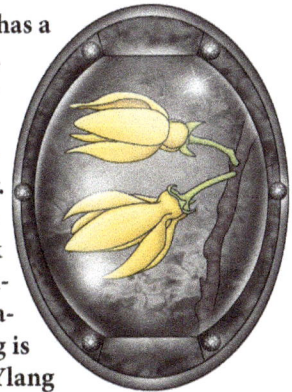

Ylang Ylang

11

"Forgiveness"

Using essential oils in a diffuser is considered one of the safest and effective ways to experience aroma-therapy, which makes it a preferred method for take home remedies. Just a few drops of essential oil can deliver a fine vapor throughout the room and can be easily absorbed via the respiratory system. Since heat can cause essential oils to degrade quickly, cold or ultrasonic diffusion is preferred to obtain full thera-peutic effects. Do not use Soldiers Stories Unwound elixirs and essential oils in a nebulizer.

Home Remedies

In a large diffuser, place 20 drops of Forgiveness elixir in a full well of filtered or purified water. Run diffuser 1 hour before retiring, either on constant or interval setting. Repeat daily or nightly until both provider and patient are ready for the next elixir of Soldiers Stories Unwound.

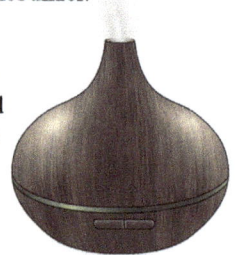

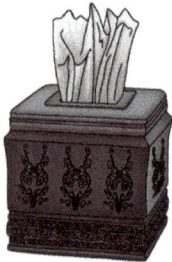

Drip 10 drops of Forgiveness elixir on a tissue. Slip tissue under the pillow case and inhale as you sleep. Repeat nightly until both provider and patient are ready for the next elixir.

Have patient assume a comfortable, meditative posture while taking a few deep breaths. Repeat the following phrases, like a mantra, for 7 to 8 times. "I'm sorry, Please forgive me, Thank you, I love you". Take time to reflect and breath after repeating the phrases. This simple practice of Ho'oponopono requires both attention and intention. When done correctly, it is said to be one of the most freeing experiences.

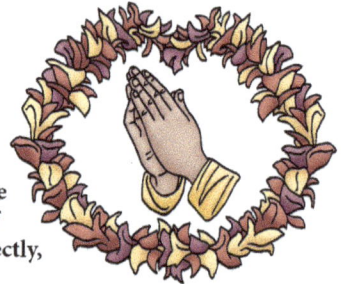

Ho'oponopono is an ancient spiritual practice that involves taking responsibility for everything around us. It means to "set things right" or "back into balance". This prayer is a tool for restoring self-love and balance. Chanting this prayer is a powerful way to cleanse the body of guilt, shame, haunting memories, ill will or bad feelings that keep the mind fixated on negative thoughts.

12

"Self-Reflection"

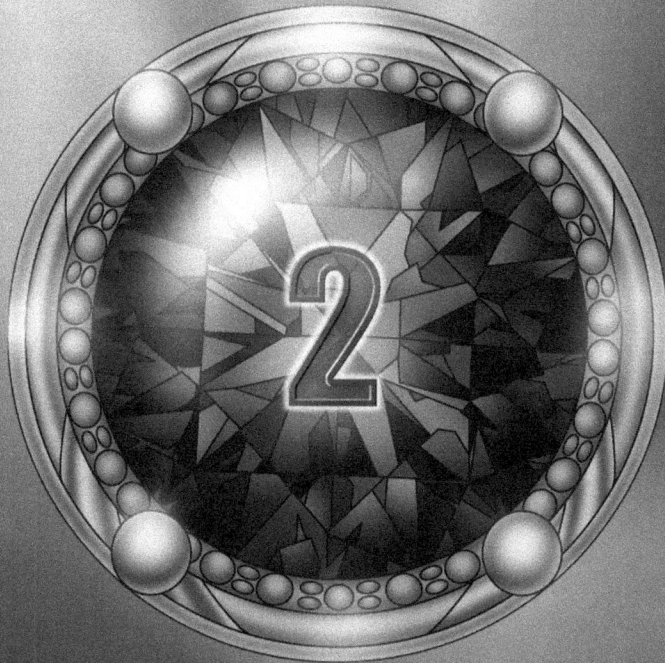

2

SOLDIERS STORIES UNWOUND

"Self-Reflection"

Self-Reflection is the second protocol and is used upon the completion of the Forgiveness protocol. The old adage, "what you resist, persists" comes into play here. Many symptoms become more intense when we resist feelings and issues that come up to the surface. Self-Reflection encourages the veteran to gently face these feelings and issues with clarity. This protocol is charged on the Flower of Life grid with the snowflake obsidian stone. This is the gentlest of the confrontational obsidian stones and is "designed" to help us face ourselves clearly with compassion. This allows the veteran to see where improvement needs to occur and what issues need addressing. The Diamond Gem Elixir is used here, due to the diamond gem's pure white and full spectral light. It amplifies the functions of the obsidian stone and essential oils in this elixir. It creates clarity and sparkle, the seed of life.

Self-Reflection Elixir In Camanu Carrier Oil

Ingredients: Ylang Ylang, Damask Rose Neet, Blue Tansy, Bergamot, Neroli, Coriander Seed, Holy Basil, Rosemary, Black Pepper, Sweet Orange, Grand Fir Essential Oils and Diamond Gem Elixir. Elixir is charged 30 minutes on the Flower of Life grid with the snowflake obsidian stone. This is done in nature on a sunny morning around 8am.

"Self-Reflection"

Aroma Acupoint Protocol

Throughout our lives, there are instances where we temporarily push down feelings so we can continue with our everyday living. This couldn't be more true of veterans in battle, who bury these intense life experiences in the interest of survival. After time, many of these buried life experiences show up as symptoms of pain, anxiety and more. This 2nd protocol, Self-Reflection, supports the process of bringing these experiences to light in a gentle and meaningful way. This protocol can be administered through direct contact, galaxy cotton ball or double tipped cotton stick method. See pages 52 and 53. The direct contact method is used below. Start with patient in a supine position, arms at their sides with palms facing up. Consider asking the patient to breath into the space with the most tension to encourage important information to emerge. Be prepared to refer patients who need support with this process.

1. YinTang - Seated at the head of the patient, put 1 drop of Self-Reflection blend on one finger or galaxy cotton swab. Place lightly over the "third eye" and hold for 1 minute or longer, until a shift occurs. This could be a deep breath from the patient, an unwinding of energy, etc...

2. Anmian - Reapply 1-2 drops of blend on index finger and transfer to finger of your second hand by pressing them together lightly. Seated at the head of your patient, slide your hands face up to place fingers with essential oil behind their ears. Hold lightly on both points for 1 minute or until a shift occurs.

3. HT6 - Repeat application of Self-Reflection to both fingers as above. Standing at the side of your patient, lightly place blend on patient's inside arms, close to wrist on the ulner side. Again, hold lightly until shift occurs, about 1 minute.

Yintang

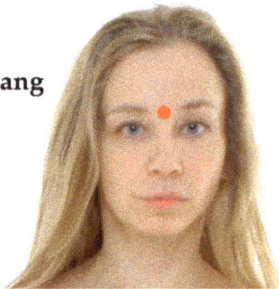

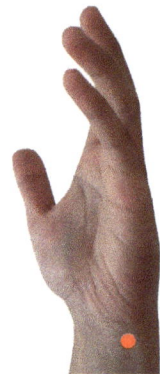

HT 6

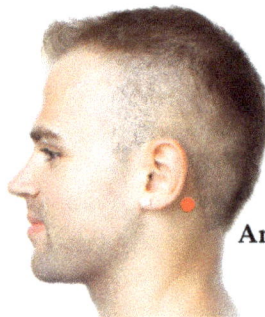

Anmian

"Self-Reflection"

Point Location and Functions

Yin Tang - Hall of Seal - Midway between the medial ends of the eyebrows. Dispels wind-heat, calms the spirit, addresses insomnia, anxiety and stress; frontal headache, sinusitis and congestion. Increases intuition and self awareness. The main focus of this protocol is to calm the spirit and increase self awareness, but can address many other symptoms as well.

Anmian - Peaceful Sleep - The midpoint between TH17 and GB20. (TH17 is posterior to lobule of the ear, in the depression between the mandible and the mastoid process. GB20 is located in a depression between the upper portion of the sternocleidomastoid muscle (SCM) and the trapezius, level with GV16).Primarily addresses insomnia and dream disturbed sleep; but also vertigo, headache, palpitations and mental disorders.

HT6 - Yin Xi/Yin Cleft - When the palm faces upward, the point is located on the radial side of the flexor carpi ulnaris tendon, .5 cun above the wrist crease on the line between HT3 and HT7.

Counterflow of qi, including panic attacks, nosebleeds; acute emotional disturbances, including mania, anxiety, shock and sudden loss of voice. This point addresses night sweats and chest/heart pain from blood stasis.

"Self-Reflection"

Essences and Their Functions

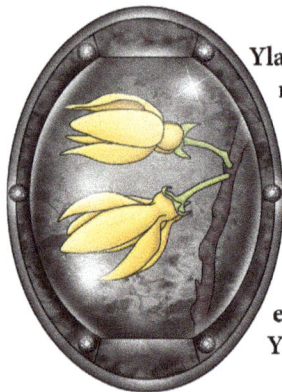

Ylang Ylang (*Cananga odorata*) is used here in Self-Reflection because of it's regulatory function, specifically of an overstimulated nervous system. It's name means "flower of flowers" and it has a sweet, sensual scent that can be described as euphoric. This allows the recipient to feel safe in uncovering whatever emerges in their self evaluation. It's uplifting effect relieves depression and increases self-esteem. Ylang Ylang is predominantly associated with the Heart and addresses anxiety, tension, palpitations, anger and insomnia, as well as shock or trauma. The stabilizing effect on moods and emotions is the main reason Ylang Ylang is used here Ylang Ylang 1 from Madagascar is the oil extraction used in this blend.

Ylang Ylang

Damask Rose (*Rosa damascena*) - neet - Damask Rose has an affinity with the heart and connects us to divine source. Rose's sweet aromatic scent not only softens the hardened heart, it also nourishes the heart. Rose essential oil imparts compassionate acceptance of self and helps resolve feelings of shame and anger turned inward and other feelings that contribute to self sabotage. It heals the heart damaged by these feelings, as well as by patterns of domination, submission and abuse. This leaves the recipient supported in their endeavor of self reflection. Rose helps with mood swings, low self-esteem, anxiety, depression, jealousy and envy because of it's balancing, calming and nurturing effects. Rose Essential oil is obtained via steam distillation of organic blossoms of Rosa Damascena from Bulgaria.

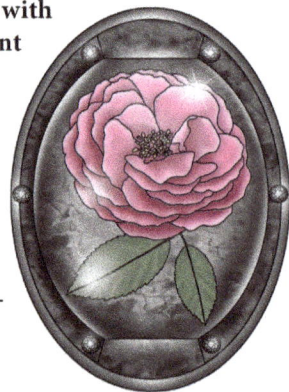

Damask Rose

"Self-Reflection"

Essences and Their Functions

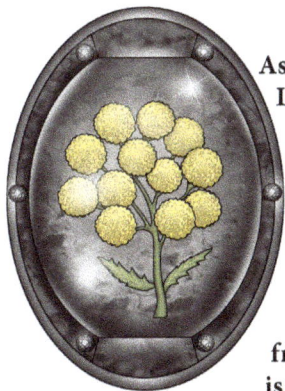

Blue Tansy

As Damask Rose has an affinity to the heart, so too has Blue Tansy to the Liver and Pericardium. Blue Tansy (*Tanacetum annuum*) is very direct and allows us to see ourselves clearly, but with joy and humor. These attributes allow the smooth flow of the emotions and softening around the heart to occur as self reflection takes place. It relieves feelings of frustration, irritability, anger and oversensitivity, as well as eases stress, tension, anxiety and worry. It's sweet green aspect harmonizes as the spicy undertones uplift and the fruity aspect brings sweetness to the experience. The essential oil is extracted from the fresh Moroccan herb and flowering buds by steam distillation. It's color is a deep marine blue due to it's Chamazulene content which brings joy and a feeling of calm.

Bergamot (*Citrus bergamia*) balances the right and left brain, bringing the logical and creative attributes into harmony. It expands and opens perspectives, allowing higher truths to emerge and internal conflicts to resolve. This is the underlying purpose of this blend! Additionally, it clears agitation, calms the heart and brings balance to the central nervous system, providing a strong foundation for integration of any resolutions. It is uplifting, and relieves depression, nervousness and insomnia. Bergamot is obtained through a cold extraction of unripe bergamot fruit rinds. The color is light emerald or olive green with a warm fruity, sweet aroma with fresh citrus overtones. Bergamot is photo sensitizing which could cause irritations and burns if exposed to the sun.

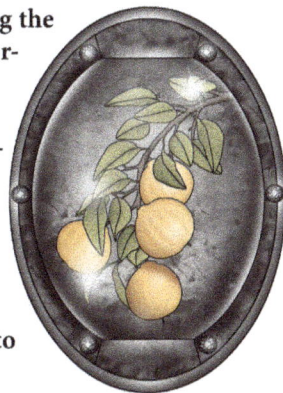

Bergamot

19

"Self-Reflection"

Essences and Their Functions

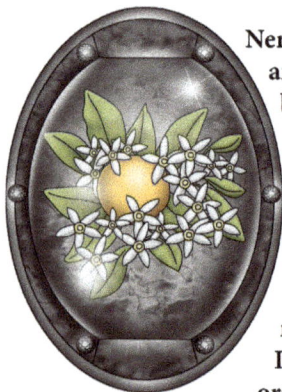

Neroli

Neroli (*Citrus aurantium*) - Neroli is like being kissed by an angel, so light and ethereal... and divine, because the feeling stays with you. Neroli is beneficial on many levels. It is the most stabilizing of the flower essences and instills will power, the ability to focus, and healthy boundaries. It is included in this blend for these attributes, and also it's effects on unproductive guilt. The mind-body can get stuck in loops of guilt and shame. Neroli can gently move this energy, while at the same time engender a safe and integrated self. Other benefits include relieving digestive disorders caused by anxiety or fear, regulating the rhythm of the heart and encouraging heart opening, bringing in joy. It's essential oil is extracted from the flower blossoms of the bitter orange tree of Italy.

Coriander Seed (*Coriandrum sativum*) - Coriander, the herb, is used in many of our kitchens and is recognized as food. As such, coriander seed essential oil is used here to nourish and fill our mind-body. Physically, it helps digestion and transforms dampness. Emotionally, this essential oil fulfills spaces of lack or less than. This includes feelings of abandonment, insecurity and bitterness, which may constrict the throat. Here coriander helps us find our voice and speak our truth. Coriander seed can also alleviate feelings of hopelessness, worry, shock and fear as we feel supported from the inside, from our own power, trusting our own bodies to heal. Extracted from the seed, this essential oil connects us to earth and to our birth right of abundance and personal potential. This essential oil originates from Poland.

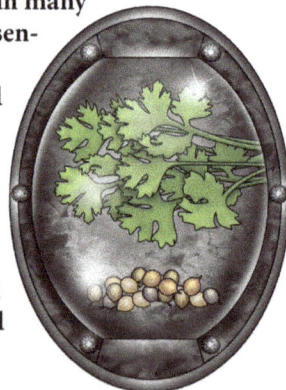

Coriander Seed

20

Essences and Their Functions

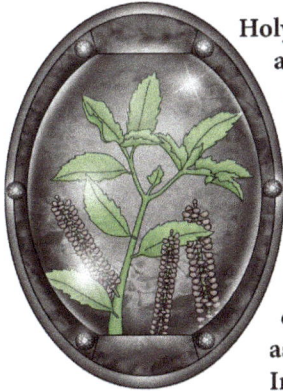

Holy Basil (*Ocimum sanctum*) is considered a purifier of the mind, body, and spirit. Holy basil, also known as Tulsi, has a special place in Hindu courtyards across India, where it is planted for its auspicious and protective powers. Scientifically, it is described as an adaptogen that manages cellular stress and acts as an adrenal restorative. It has a licorice, mint-like aroma which can be diffused to help promote sleep, as well as calm the mind. Known for its mental and spiritual awakening properties, Holy Basil increases concentration as it eases muscle tension. It is an anti-inflammatory, antidepressant, antiviral oil which contains cholesterol-lowering properties, relieves pain, acts as a digestive aid, and supports the thyroid. This essential oil from India is extracted through steam distillation.

Holy Basil

Rosemary (*Rosmarinus officinalis*) essential oil is extracted from the fresh leafy shrub in flower via steam distillation. This oil from Spain is clear with a green herbaceous aroma and has a fresh pungent energetic. It's uplifting nature addresses feelings of lethargy, apathy and low self-esteem. It helps one lead from the heart, perfect in cases of withdrawal, detachment and other forms of disconnection. Rosemary is indicated in cardiac, respiratory, digestive, liver and uterine weaknesses. As such, the essential oil is contraindicated during pregnancy and in cases of hypertension. It is used here for it's warm, stimulating and restorative nature which enhances concentration and motivation. Rosemary also treats the psychological disorders of ADD and depression.

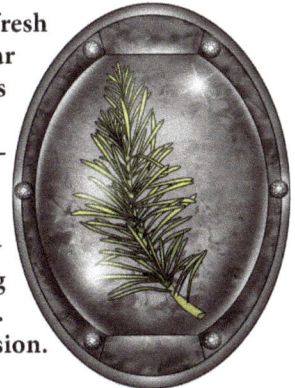

Rosemary

"Self-Reflection"

Essences and Their Functions

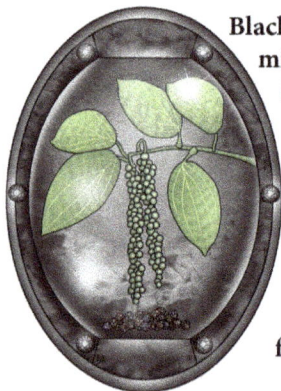

Black Pepper (*Piper nigrum*) is another one of those kitchen herbs that remind the body of home and nourishment. As such, it aids digestion and is easily assimilated. The essential oil is warm, stimulating and invigorating which is perfect for states of lethargy, depression and especially, cold indifference. It's action of resolving damp can help unearth trapped memories and traumas in the body, bringing them to the forefront for examination. Black pepper is used in this blend to do just that, while encouraging one to take action. This oil is clear and pungent with a fresh, spicy aroma with woody, rooty undertones. This Black Pepper essential oil is from Madagascar and is extracted from the dried peppercorns through steam distillation.

Black Pepper

Sweet Orange (*Citrus aurantium*) has a name that brings back images of childhood and is used to treat the younger ones as a rule. It's presence in this essential oil blend is to bring back the innocence and joy of an earlier time in order to regain trust in playfulness and spontaneity, while eradicating thoughts and behaviors that are controlling, overly serious and cynical. Sweet Orange essential oil helps us to redirect love and acceptance to our shadow side, the aspects of self that we reject and prefer to remain hidden. It's uplifting, harmonizing and balancing attributes help to regulate mood, settle the heart and harmonize the spirit. Sweet orange essential oil is extracted via cold press of the organic orange rinds from South Africa.

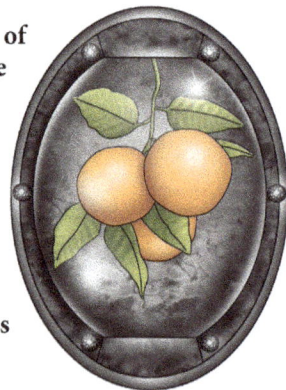

Sweet Orange

22

Essences and Their Functions

Grand Fir (*Abies grandis*) invokes wisdom as conifers are ancient beings. Grand Fir has been used for centuries by Native Americans who steeped the fresh needles in hot water to make teas and baths. Early shamans used the needles of the Grand Fir to purify the skin before religious ceremonies. Many tribes even burned the needles and inhaled the smoke to clear their bodies and minds, especially the lungs. It's clarifying aspect aids the mind in focusing, freeing it from distractions. Grand Fir can also relieve suffering from fatigue, anxiety, and depression by elevating the mood. The essential oil is restoring and motivating, which discourages withdrawal and encourages connection. This oil from France is extracted via steam distillation of the end twigs and needles.

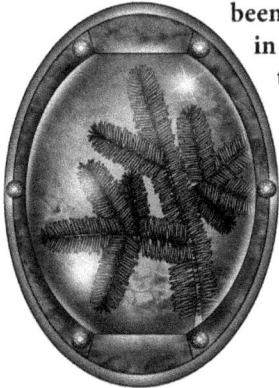

Grand Fir

The hardest stone, the Diamond (*Diamas*) produces the sharpest refractive colors, giving your body clarity and sparkle. Called the king of gemstones, diamond cuts away impurities, imparting a sense of transparency to one's field. It's crystalline nature opens and balances the cranial plates in the head, helping them to breathe and transmit light to the rest of your body. The Diamond Elixir clears emotional and mental pain, reduces fear and brings about new beginnings. It aids spiritual evolution and reminds you of your soul's aspirations. Diamond Elixir brings clarity to your thoughts and feelings by purifying and aligning your body at cellular levels. This elixir is made by placing gems in a bowl of purified water in early morning sunlight.

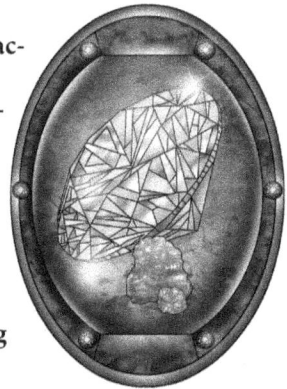

23

Diamond Elixir

"Self-Reflection"

Self-Reflection Blend was charged on the circle of life grid with a Snowflake Obsidian stone. A stone of purity, Snowflake Obsidian brings about balance to body, mind and spirit. It can remove negativity from a space or person with ease. Obsidian is molten lava that cools so quickly that theres no time for crystallization to occur. Volcanic in nature, this stone helps draw emotions up to the surface to be examined in relationship with harmful thought patterns. It's truth enhancing, reflective qualities are merciless in exposing flaws, weakness and blockages. Having said that, Snowflake Obsidian calms and soothes, putting you in the right frame of mind to be receptive before bringing your attention to ingrained patterns of behavior. It has no boundaries or limitations, so it works extremely fast and with great power to bring truth to the surface to be resolved. Snowflake Obsidian teaches us to value mistakes as well as successes.

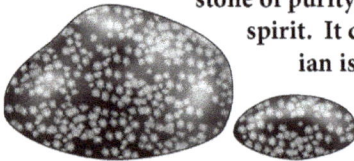

Snowflake Obsidian

Home Remedy

As was stated previously, diffusing essential oils is one of the safest and beneficial methods of aromatherapy. The aroma can prompt the nervous system to transmit signals to the limbic system in the brain, the same part of the brain that houses emotion and memory. The brain may respond by initiating various physiological functions, such as hormone release, pain relief, or a positive boost in mood. This elixir can be used in ultrasonic diffusers. Do not use in a nebulizer.

In a large diffuser, place 15 drops of Self-Reflection elixir in a full well of filtered or purified water. Run diffuser 1 hour before retiring, either on constant or interval setting. Repeat nightly until both provider and patient are ready for the next elixir of Soldiers Stories Unwound.

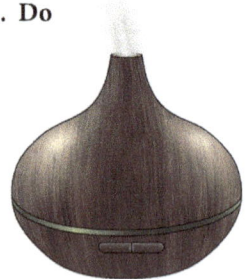

"Back From the Darkness"

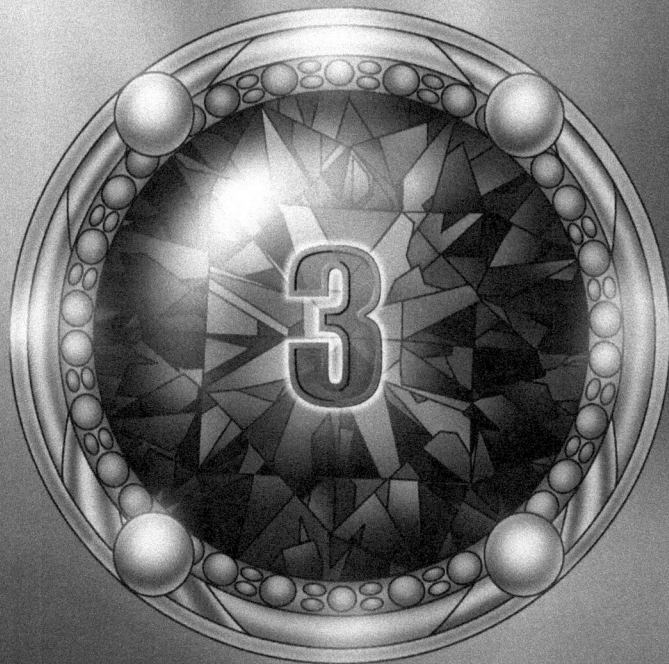

3

SOLDIERS STORIES UNWOUND

"Back from the Darkness"

Back From the Darkness gently brings painful and repressed feelings to the surface. It allows them to be acknowledged and then dissipated through emotional release. Secondly and compassionately, this third elixir opens the heart and allows playfulness to enter back into one's life. It imparts a vitality and affinity to happiness that is divine. It lifts a depressed mood and brings lightness into life and satisfies a longing for spirit. This elixir contains alcohol for preservation and color therapy. In cases of addiction, or for other objections to alcohol, I have included a crystal protocol that can serve as a great alternative to the elixir.

Back From The Darkness Elixir In Purified Water

Ingredients: Rhodochrosite Elixir, Blue Lotus Flower Essence and Blue Curaçao.
Rhodochrosite Elixir charged on Flower of Life grid in sunlight.

Rhodochrosite, Merlinite and Uvarovite Garnet crystal protocol. Place Rhodochrosite on the midline of the chest, close to the heart (CV17); Merlinite is placed on the notch of the neck on the midline of the body (above CV22); and Garnet is placed on the third eye in center of the forehead (Yintang). Optimally, the protocol should remain on these points for one hour in the evening before retiring.

"Back from the Darkness"

Aroma Acupoint Protocol

This protocol continues the process of releasing traumatic experiences and feelings within the mind-body, while awakening to the realization of true self and all it's possibilities. It lifts the darkness of negative thoughts and fears to reveal the full spectrum of life, with joy and vitality. This protocol can be administered through direct contact, galaxy cotton ball or double tipped cotton stick method shown on pages 52 and 53. The direct contact method is described below. Start with the patient in a supine position, with arms at the sides.

Sishencong - Sit at the head of the patient. Place 1-2 drops on the thumb and index finger of one of your hands and transfer to second hand by lightly pressing the thumb and index fingers of both hands together. Gently place all four digits on crown of patient's head, the four points of sishencong. Hold lightly until shift occurs, about 1-2 minutes.

SP21 - Continue treatment by having the patient put their hands behind their head, cradling their head like a pillow, in the supine position. Standing at the side of patient, place 1-2 drops of elixir on the index finger of one hand and lightly make contact with index finger of the other hand to transfer elixir. Gently hold index fingers with elixir to SP21 on both sides of the torso. Hold until a shift occurs, about 1 minute.

PC8 - Have patient place their arms down at their sides, with palms facing up. Add 1-2 drops of elixir to the index fingers as described above. Gently hold index fingers on Lao Gong, PC8, on both hands of patient for 1 minute or until a shift occurs.

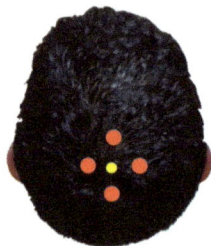

● = Sishencong

● = GV 20 as reference point

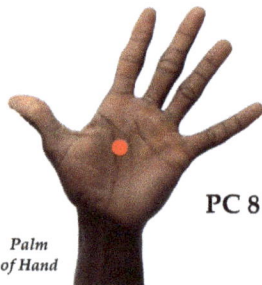

PC 8

*Palm
of Hand*

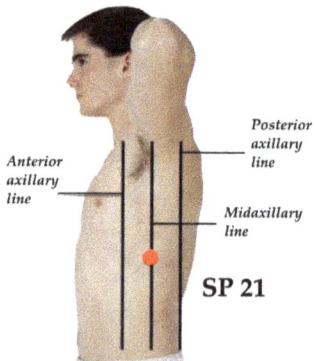

*Posterior
axillary
line*

*Anterior
axillary
line*

*Midaxillary
line*

SP 21

"Back from the Darkness"

Point Location and Functions

Sishencong/God's Cleverness or Alert Spirit Quartet - A group of four points at the crown of the head, 1 cun bilateral, posterior and anterior to GV20. Pacifies wind and calms the spirit, useful for epilepsy, wind stroke, headache, and vertigo. Treatment with these points improves relaxation and addresses insomnia, memory loss and ADHD.

Spleen 21 - Dabao/Great Embracement - Bilaterally located on the lateral side of the torso, on the mid-axillary line in the 6th intercostal space, approximately 6 cun below the axilla. As the Great Luo, SP21 is connected to all the organ systems of the body via the luo channels, and therefore treats the entire body. The emotional/spiritual function of this point is likened to an existential hug or embrace. Treatment of this point addresses flaccid joints, thoracic pain, or pain all over the body. It descends Lung Qi which addresses conditions of cough, asthma, chest oppression and shortness of breath.

Pericardium 8 - Lao Gong/Palace of Toil - Bilaterally located on the transverse crease of the palm, between the 2nd and 3rd metacarpal bones. When a loose fist is made, it is located where the tip of the middle finger falls. This point is used with this blend for it's dual function of easing anxiety and clearing inflammation. Treatment of this point cools the Heart and clears heat, including heat in the blood. Emotionally, this point clears the heat and bitterness of anger which obstructs the pathway to joy. In addition to clearing the pathway for joy, PC8 addresses cardiac pain, mental disorders, epilepsy, gastritis, foul breath and bleeding due to heat; which includes blood in the urine and stool, plus nosebleeds. This point can also be used for fungus infection of the hand and foot, nausea and vomiting. It's location on the open palm of the hand, allows this point to be extremely receptive to healing.

Essences and Their Functions

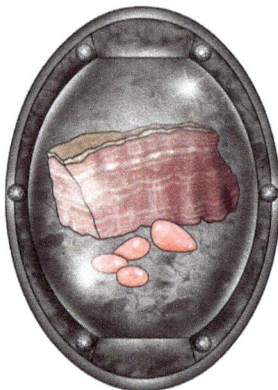

Rhodochrosite Elixir

The crystal rhodochrosite is pink to orange and represents selfless love and compassion. Rhodochrosite (a manganese carbonate mineral) is an excellent stone for the heart and relationships, especially for people who feel unloved. It is the stone par excellence for healing sexual abuse. This stone continues the process of tackling one's issues as rhodochrosite gently brings painful and repressed feelings to the surface to be acknowledged and emotionally released, without shutting down. This stone insists you face the truth, about yourself and others, without excuses or evasion, but with loving awareness. Rhodochrosite imparts a dynamic and positive attitude. It improves self worth and soothes emotional stress.

Blue Lotus (*Nymphaea caerula*) is described as the world's highest vibrational flower. Native to India and Egypt, this beautiful and mysterious flower is actually a water lily and not a true lotus. One of the most illusive and sought after flowers, Blue Lotus's sublime aroma imparts high levels of energy and divine feelings of mystical love. In addition, this essence creates the awareness of life as divine play. Blue Lotus imparts vitality and happiness to the full spectrum of your mind, body and spirit and brings the sublime to everyday life. No other vibrational substance reaches as deeply into the cellular level and satisfies a longing for spirit as does Blue Lotus. This flower, made as an essence on the Big Island, is a gift from Hawaii as it was located in the most unforeseen, miraculous way.

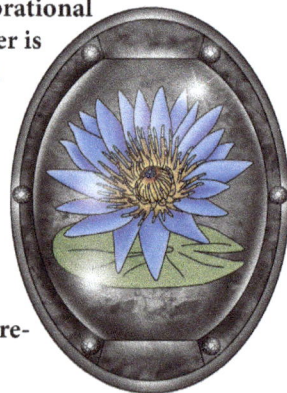

Blue Lotus Essence

"Back from the Darkness"

Below are 2 remedies that can be practiced at home. The first remedy contains a small amount of alcohol, so if there is an objection to ingesting alcohol, please suggest the 2nd protocol, a crystal treatment, which requires 3 crystals or mineral stones.

Home Remedies

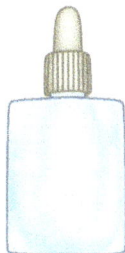

Oral therapy - 2 to 3 drops of Back from the Darkness elixir, 3 times a day under the tongue until 15 ml bottle is finished.

Crystal therapy - Collect the crystals rhodochrosite, merlinite, garnet and place within reach. While veteran lies face up, in a supine position, place rhodochrosite over the heart center or CV17. Then place merlinite in the throat indentation, between CV22 and CV23. The garnet crystal can be placed on the forehead between the eyebrows or "third eye", YinTang. I recommend the uvarovite garnet for this protocol. Below are some characteristics and functions of these crystals.

Rhodochrosite - As previously mentioned, rhodochrosite imparts a positive attitude and selfless compassion. It soothes emotional stress, while facing the truth about yourself and others.
Merlinite - As the name implies, merlinite can bring magic into your life. It can heal past lives and brings harmony into the present life. It balances masculine and feminine energies, yin/yang, the conscious and subconscious, as well as the intellect and intuition.
Uvarovite Garnet - Garnet is a powerful stone with a myriad of healing qualities and functions. A regenerating stone, garnet revitalizes, purifies, and balances energy, bringing serenity or passion where appropriate. The uvarovite garnet is a calm and peaceful stone. It promotes individuality without egocentricity. It is stimulating to the heart chakra and enhances spiritual relationships.

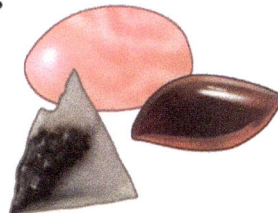

31

"Silver Lining"

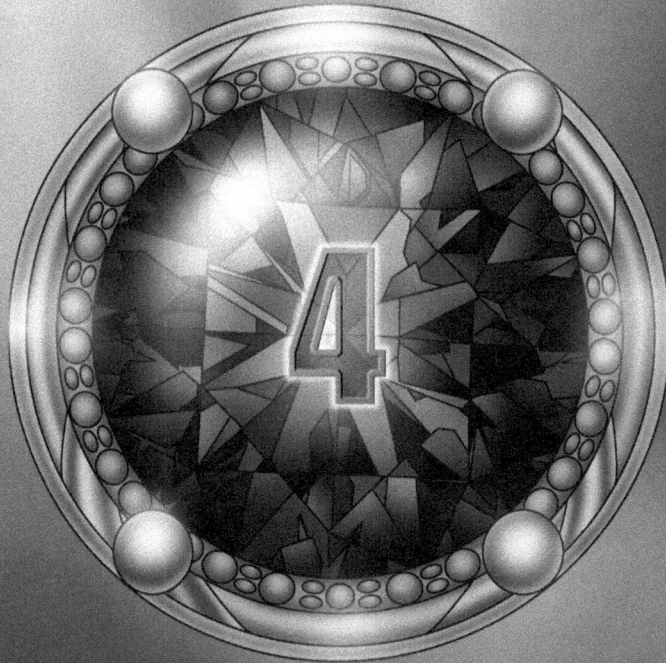

4

SOLDIERS STORIES UNWOUND

"Silver Lining"

Personal growth is the silver lining that comes with hardship. The third elixir allows the veteran to return to self and at a higher vibration. This fourth elixir, Silver Lining, aids in the veteran's reconnection to the outside world; both established relationships, as well as new contacts.

The Silver Lining protocol, includes treatment of individual acupuncture points, coupled with a back treatment, including the spine. The spine houses the central nervous system, which is greatly affected by stress. This elixir contains essential oils that aid in calming the energetic "buzz" that accumulates along the spine due to stress response. Black Spruce, included in this blend, is the essential oil *par excellence* to treat this accumulation.

Silver Lining allows the veteran to let go of old armoring, possibly guilt and shame, to regain trust and joy, in order to live a life of fulfillment free from past traumas.

Silver Lining Elixir in Jojoba Carrier Oil

Ingredients: Black Spruce, Coriander Seed, Jasmine Sambac, Mandarin, Marjoram, and Neroli.

Compounded using Rose Quartz and Rhodochrosite Gem Stone.

"Silver Lining"

Aroma Acupoint Protocol

This protocol reaches deeper into the crevices of the mind-body. It touches the organ systems, clears the channels, soothes the spirit and pacifies the heart. It encourages recognition of one's connection to others and it's vibrational effects. This elixir is useful in easing a hyperactive, fixed sympathetic response to a more restorative, parasympathetic one. It can be useful in conditions of ADHD, panic attacks, anxiety and more. This protocol is best administered through direct contact. See pages 52 and 53 for application techniques. Start with the patient facing down, in a prone position, arms at their sides with palms facing up.

Ht7 - Place 1-2 drops of elixir on your index finger and transfer to 2nd index finger by lightly pressing fingers together. Transfer elixir to patient's wrists at Ht7. Hold gently for 1 minute or longer until a shift occurs.

TH16 - Place 1-2 more drops of the elixir on index fingers and place on both sides of the patient's neck at TH16. Hold gently for 1 minute or longer until a shift occurs.

Back Treatment with Silver Lining Flow - Drip 5-7 drops of elixir on patient's lower back above the sacrum in lumbar dip. Then drip elixir about every 3 inches up the Huatuojiaji line (L5-T1) on left side of body and then down the right Huatuojiaji line. Continue the drip up the center spine or Governing Vessel to shoulders and down the outer Urinary Bladder line on the right side of body and up the outer Urinary Bladder line on left side of body. Place 1 to 2 fingers in the small pool of elixir above the patient's sacrum and make a small circle there and follow the same pathway of the drip sequence outlined above, finishing down the center spine to repeat sequence. Repeat slowly for a total of three passes, ending at C7/T1. Cover patient's back with sheet or milar blanket for at least 5 minutes, preferably longer.

"Silver Lining"

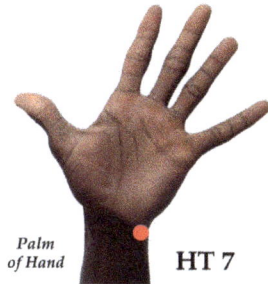

Palm of Hand — HT 7

TH 16

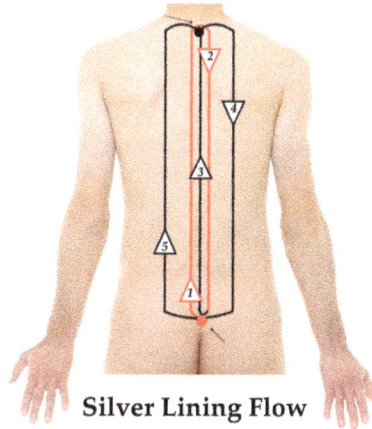

Silver Lining Flow

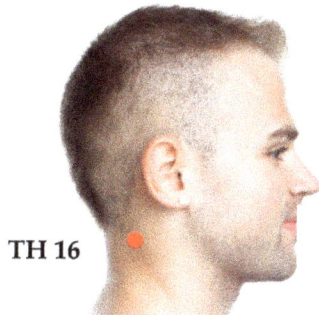

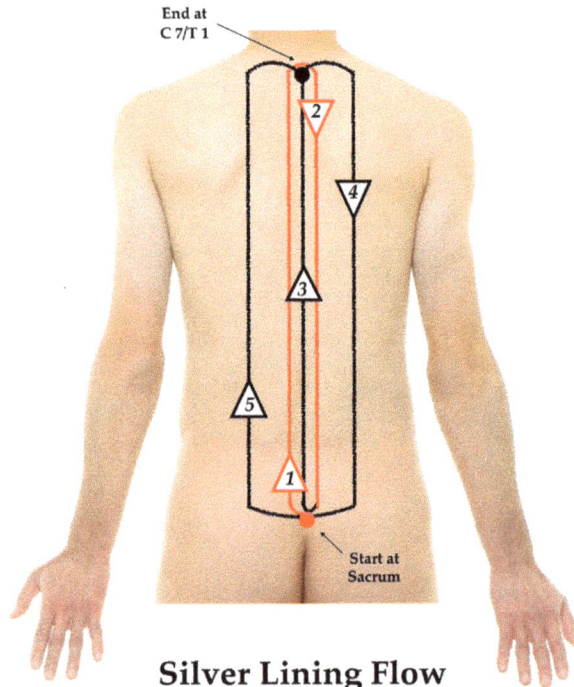

End at C 7/T 1

Start at Sacrum

Silver Lining Flow

Using Outer Bladder Meridian, Governing Vessel & Huátúojiājǐ Points

"Silver Lining"

Point Location and Functions

Ht7 - Shen Men/Spirit Gate - This point is located on the inside wrist crease, on the radial side of the flexor carpi ulnaris tendon, between the ulna and pisiform bones. This point is used here for it's affinity with physical responses to emotional stimuli; ie, anxiety with palpitations, nausea with panic and/or fear. Any emotional response that gets in the way from enjoying a life of trust and joy. It also addresses insomnia and muddled thinking.

TH16 - Tianyou/Celestial Pillar or Window - Find this point directly below the mastoid process level with the mandibular angle and on the posterior border of the SCM muscle. Located in line with SI17 and GV15. This point is mentioned in Chapter 21 of the Ling Shu and it's usage in treating an abrupt loss of hearing. Celestial Pillar also falls into the category of Window of the Sky points that were developed by Dr. Chamfrault and Dr. Van Nghi in 1954. Practitioners use this point in a number of capacities, but this point is used here for it's connecting function to one's spiritual self and also for its aid in releasing emotional trauma from both current and past life experiences.

Silver Lining Flow - This back treatment follows the pathways of 2 major meridians as well as the path of the Huatojiaji. The first and second pathways follow a vertical line connecting the huatuojiaji, which are a group of 34 points located .5 cun (about 1/2") bilaterally from the lower border of each spinous process from T1 to L5. Traditionally, these points are used to treat the upper and lower limbs, the chest and abdomen according to the location of enervation. The next pathway is up the center spine or Governing Vessel meridian. The treatment follows a small portion of this meridian from the top of the sacrum up to where the spine meets the neck. The last pathway is the Urinary Bladder Meridian that runs 3 cun (or inches) from the center spine or Governing Vessel. This meridian includes the Back Shu points that have a direct pathway to the vital organs.

"Silver Lining"

Essences and Their Functions

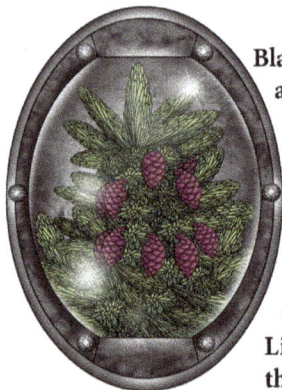

Black Spruce

Black Spruce (*Picea marinara*) has an intimate relationship with personal growth as is it's function in this elixir. This is best described by it's transformational relationship with fire. Although this majestic tree is not impervious to forest fire, it can survive one. It's crown of cones that house the seeds, located high in its branches, can avoid the destructive flames. And it's potential can be realized through the planting of these seeds in the ashes. Like a phoenix rising from the ashes, black spruce seedlings rise up again to fulfill it's destiny. This transformational quality is imparted to the recipient of this Silver Lining elixir; the death or letting go of the old self, so that a more authentic self can emerge. Black Spruce's restorative and regulative nature of the neuroendocrine-immune system is also paramount to this elixir.

Coriander Seed (*Coriandrum sativum*) is welcomed by the human body because of it's familiarity as food from our kitchens. It's nourishing properties remind us of hearth and home bringing a level of comfort and nourishment to the recipient. It's ability to satisfy and fill the empty spaces in the mind-body are aspects that make this essential oil irreplaceable in this blend. This essential oil embraces the whole of our being, reminding us to tap into our own resources, including our intuition, directing us on our path in life and healing. It's lemony aspect is uplifting, while it's green herbal quality is harmonizing. Coming from a seed, this essence imparts the ability to digest life experience, paving the way for the future. Coriander seed addresses mental/emotional conditions of anxiety, depression, hopelessness, and nervous exhaustion.

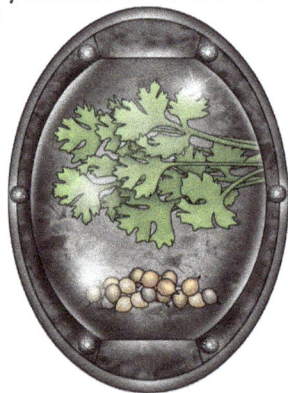

Coriander Seed

"Silver Lining"

Essences and Their Functions

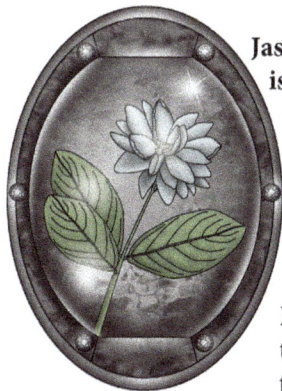

Jasmine sambac (*Jasminum sambac*) is an essential oil with depth. It is cool, with a sweet-green and sweet-floral aroma with lyrical top notes. The plant is often called "Queen of the Night" as it mysteriously blooms in the evening hours and has an alluring fragrance. It's relationship with the darkness helps the recipient of this oil face the darker side of themselves and their circumstances in life. Simultaneously, it helps heal trauma and shock which makes facing the difficult possible, as it is uplifting, euphoric and calming. It releases constraint around the heart, allowing it to open up and trust where trust was lost. Jasmine sambac heals guilt and shame that can arise with sexual violations, allowing trust of the body to also occur.

Jasmine Sambac

Mandarin, Red (*Citrus aurantium*) essential oil is extracted from the rind of the ripened fruit. It's aroma is sweet-lemony and is uplifting, clarifying, harmonizing while relaxing. It has a fresh, tangy profile that mixes bright citrus with sweet, fruity heart notes. It's simplicity and directness engenders pure joy, innocence and honesty in general. It is a favorite of children and the inner child in all of us. It's cheering, uplifting and relaxing aroma is ideal for treating negative emotional conditions such as anxiety, nervous tension, stress, irritability, restlessness and tantrums at any age. Its strong circulatory and diuretic functions make it effective in reducing phlegm and treating fluid retention. This essential oil is also helpful in relieving dyspepsia and gastritis.

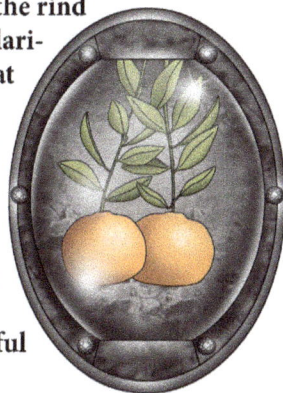

39

Mandarin

"Silver Lining"

Essences and Their Functions

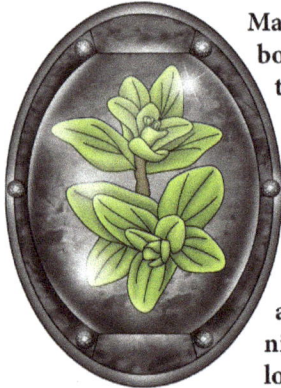

Marjoram (*Origanum maiorana*) is a dual action essential oil as it has both relaxant and restorative properties. This sweet-herbaceous essential oil relaxes the mind/body/spirit. Emotionally, it relaxes automatic resistance to inside or outside stimuli, as it also restores healthy boundaries without undo influence of the past. Physically, marjoram relaxes the armature of the muscle body, including the heart muscle, facilitating the release of traumatic muscle memories that no longer serve. Marjoram is used in this blend for it's calming, cooling and balancing effects for the soul, while providing relaxing, warming and antispasmodic qualities for the physical body. The human body recognizes this herb as food with it's long history of use in cuisine, which allows the body to be most receptive to it's effects.

Marjoram

Neroli (*Citrus aurantium*) - Neroli is like being kissed by an angel, so light and ethereal, and so divine, because the feeling stays with you. Neroli is beneficial on many levels. It is the most stabilizing of the flower essences as it instills will power, the ability to focus and create healthy boundaries. It is included in this blend for these attributes, and also it's effects on unproductive guilt. The mind-body can get stuck in loops of guilt and shame. Neroli can gently move this energy, while at the same time engender a safe and integrated self. Other benefits include relieving digestive disorders caused by anxiety or fear, regulating the rhythm of the heart and encouraging the heart to open, bringing in joy. This essential oil is extracted from the flower blossoms of the bitter orange tree of Italy.

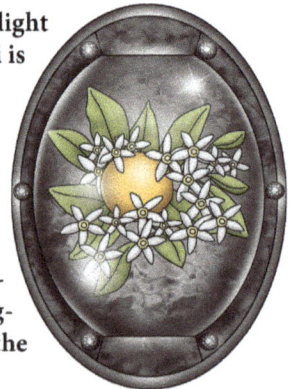

Neroli

"Silver Lining"

Essences and Their Functions

Rose Quartz is the stone of unconditional love and infinite peace. It is the most important crystal for the heart, teaching the true essence of love. It purifies and opens the heart at all levels, and brings deep inner healing and self-love. It is calming, reassuring, and excellent for use in trauma or crisis. Rose Quartz draws off negative energy and replaces it with a loving vibration. It strengthens empathy and imparts the acceptance of necessary change. Transformation is integral to Silver Lining, so acceptance of these changes is so important and is aided with the use of this gemstone. Emotionally, Rose Quartz, is the healer of unexpressed emotions and heartache, helping to release these emotions. It soothes internalized pain and heals deprivation. Rose Quartz teaches how to love yourself and invokes self-trust and self-worth.

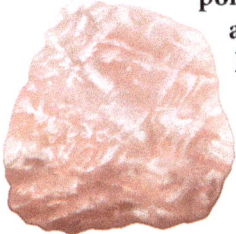

Rose Quartz

The crystal rhodochrosite is pink to orange and represents selfless love and compassion. Rhodochrosite (a manganese carbonate mineral) is an excellent stone for the heart and relationships, especially for people who feel unloved. It is the stone *par excellence* for healing sexual abuse. This stone continues the process of tackling one's issues as rhodochrosite gently brings painful and repressed feelings to the surface to be acknowledged and emotionally released, without shutting down. This stone insists you face the truth, about yourself and others, without excuses or evasion, but with loving awareness. Rhodochrosite imparts a dynamic and positive attitude. It improves self worth and soothes emotional stress.

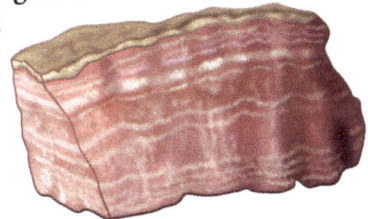

Rhodochrosite

41

"Silver Lining"

Home Remedies

Diffusing essential oils is considered one of the safest and effective ways to experience therapeutic aromatherapy. These benefits make diffusion a preferred method for take home remedies. Diffusers disperse essential oils as a fine vapor in the air so they can be absorbed gently into the body through the respiratory system. The aroma can prompt the nervous system to transmit signals to the limbic system in the brain, which may respond by initiating various physiological functions, such as a release of hormones, pain relief, or a positive boost in mood. The veteran can do one, two or all three remedies listed below.

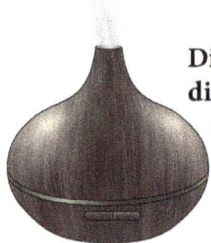

Diffusion - Add 10 drops of Silver Lining remedy to pure water in well of diffuser. Start diffusing 1 hour before retiring for a duration of one hour. Continue nightly until bottle is finished.

Spritzer- Put 5 drops of Silver Lining in 2oz of rose water in spray bottle. Spray elixir in the air and walk through droplets upon awakening. Use to encourage a calmer, more parasympathetic approach to the day.

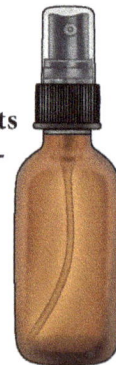

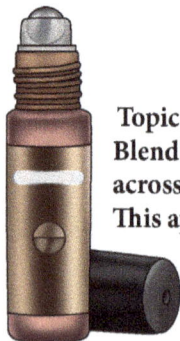

Topical Application- Upon retiring, put 1 drop of Silver Lining Blend on inner crease of wrists. If using a roll-on, do one pass across wrist. Gently hold wrists together for 1 minute or longer. This application encourages the body to enter the deep sleep stages where healing takes place and emotional debris is released.

"Peace"

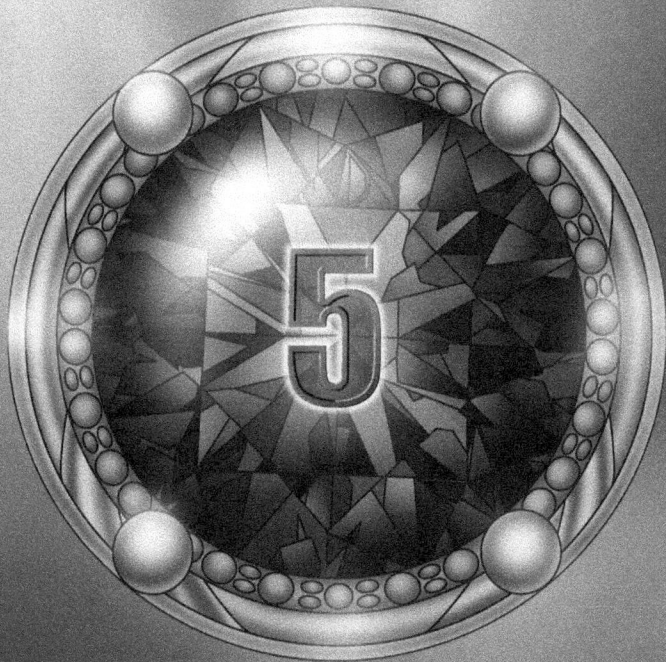

SOLDIERS STORIES UNWOUND

"Peace"

Peace is the fifth and last protocol of Soldiers Stories Unwound. As the name suggests, this elixir brings one to self, centered, and at peace. It imparts the ability to look inward, reflecting the depth and magnificence of one's true self and beauty. Part of feeling at peace is feeling safe with self and others in the outside world. On a physical level, this Peace elixir offers nurturing and immunity support, laying down a strong foundation for trust. On the emotional/spiritual level, it protects against lower vibrations as it engenders the confidence and courage to be open hearted, embracing all the beautiful things the world has to offer with a sense of humor and a positive outlook. A true homecoming.

Peace Elixir in Jojoba Carrier Oil

Ingredients: Silver Fir, Blue Tansy, Green Myrtle, Coriander Seed, and Saro Essential Oils, Silver Gem Elixir, vegetable glycerine. Peace is compounded with the vibration of Sacred Earth drum music and Property of Water bell tones. It is charged with scolecite crystal for three hours which adds a gentle, calming effect to this elixir.

"Peace"

Aroma Acupoint Protocol

This protocol works from the top of the head down to the patient's lower abdomen or center, the origin of authentic self. In Chinese medicine, this is called the Dantian, or elixir of life, where essence and spirit are stored. Traditionally, Dantian is a focal point for transmutation and is the focus in practices of qi gong, neigong, reiki and martial arts. The three Dantians refer to the energy centers at the third eye, the heart center and the lower third Dantian, treated in this protocol. Have patient lie face up on the table. Stand at the head of the patient in this supine position. The points of the protocol can be administered through direct contact, cotton galaxy or cotton stick method shown on pages 52 and 53. Direct contact method is described below.

GV20 - Transfer 2 drops of Peace elixir to your index finger and lightly place on the crown of the patient's head for 2 minutes. If you feel drawn to stay longer, place your entire palm lightly over GV20 until a shift occurs or you feel complete.

CV17 - Place 1 to 2 drops of elixir on one finger or cotton stick and gently place directly on the patient's chest or on the soft, vulnerable spot right above CV17. Hold for 1 minute or more until shift occurs.

Dantian, CV4 & GV4 - Move from the head of the patient to the patient's side. Make sure you have access to the patient's lower abdomen and lumbar spine. Put Peace elixir on your middle finger. Transfer elixir to the finger on the other hand. Carefully slide one hand under the lumbar curve of the patient and place elixir over GV4. Place finger of other hand on the lower abdomen of the patient at CV4. Hold both hands lightly as possible for 1 or more minutes until a shift occurs.

"Peace"

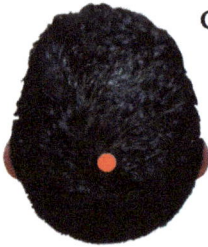

GV 20

Top of Head

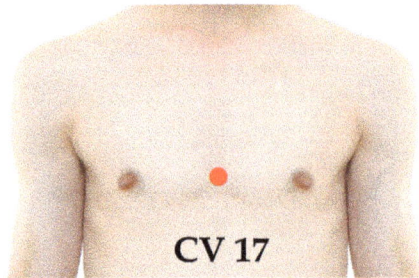

CV 17

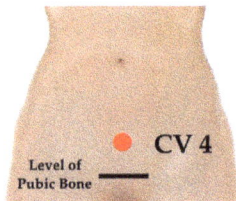

CV 4

Level of
Pubic Bone

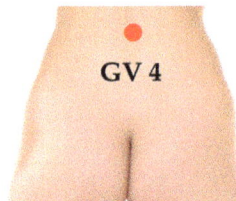

GV 4

"Peace"

Point Location and Functions

GV20 - Bai Hui/Hundred Convergences - This point is located on the crown of the head, 5 body inches posterior to the midline of the anterior hairline. It can be found at the center between the apexes of the ears or auricles. This is the first point of the three energy centers, the head, heart and dantian. Bai Hui is where the six yang channels meet with the Governing Vessel at the uppermost point of the body. In addition, it is considered the meeting place of the "hundred spirits" and is also effective in treating the "hundred diseases". It therefore is an important point to connect with spirit or Shen and address imbalances in the body. Bai Hui clears the senses, calms the spirit, dispels Liver Wind and settles Liver Yang. It can be used to treat headaches, tinnitus, nasal obstruction, vertigo, mental disorders and prolapse of the rectum or uterus.

CV17 - Dan Zhong/Chest Center - Level with the fourth intercostal space, this point is at the center of the chest, midway between the nipples. Dan Zhong is the influential point of Qi and is used here because of this function. When combined with this elixir, it connects and directs the energy between the three centers, always leading from the Heart. Dan Zhong is the main point to tonify the upper body, expanding the chest and benefitting the diaphragm. It addresses chronic lung and breast issues and guides rebellious Qi downward. This point treats conditions such as asthma, cough, shortness of breath, diaphragmatic pain, insufficient lactation and mastitis. It addresses palpitations, hiccups and difficulty swallowing.

CV4 - Guan Yuan/Origin Pass - Located on the midline of the body, 3 cun or body inches inferior to the umbilicus. This is the main point for nourishing and stabilizing the Kidneys, the seat of the Yuan Qi, while restoring the Yang and regulating Qi in the lower body.

GV4 - Ming Men/Life Gate - This point is also located on the midline of the body, below the spinous process of the second lumbar vertebra. It strengthens the Kidneys and benefits the lumbar vertebrae while nourishing the Yuan Qi. The Dantian is where this protocol ends, right where life begins, at the Life Gate. By using both CV4 and GV4 simultaneously, it brings together the future and the past, the yin and the yang, the body and the spirit into a whole, integrated self. These points combined with Peace elixir, brings the patient back to the origins, where the authentic self lives, unencumbered by the complications of life.

"Peace"

Essences and Their Functions

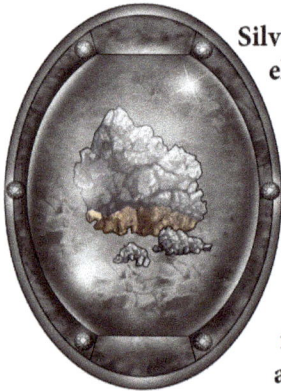

Silver Gem Elixir (*Argentum*) - The feminine, reflective aspects of this elixir helps the recipient to see themselves as they truly are, and not with any false projections. It mirrors back your true image and beauty, allowing a complete acceptance of self. Used topically, this elixir gives the body a reflective glow that deflects and gives immunity from lower vibrations. As the metal with the highest conductivity, silver works well in releasing shock or tension from the nervous system and helps the mind to process thoughts more clearly. It's antiseptic and antibacterial capacities are used in water filtration systems as a purifier. This gives a renewed sense of clarity and purity when used in baths.

Silver Gem

Silver Fir (*Abies alba*) - This essential oil brings balance, Oneness, and peace through the whole body. It helps to balance the thymus, the metabolism and serotonin levels. This balancing affect proves beneficial in relieving anxiety and stress, muscle pain and spasms, and is helpful in treating ADHD and brain integration. Silver Fir is a respiratory restorative with antimicrobial, antibiotic and antiseptic properties. The clean, fresh aroma of silver fir exerts a powerful calming influence, while at the same time providing an uplifting and refreshing feeling. Having silver in its nomenclature, brings in the reflective nature of metal. The metal element has properties of inner strength, endurance and tranquility. It has a relationship with precision and the divine.

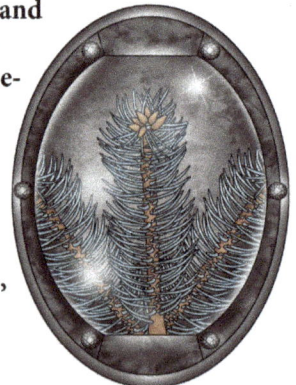

48

Silver Fir

"Peace"

Essences and Their Functions

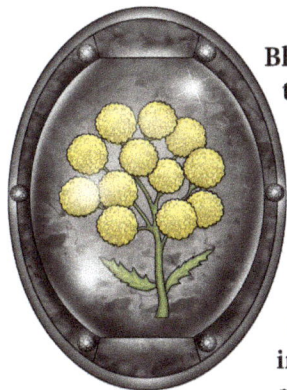

Blue Tansy (*Tanacetum annuum*) essential oil smooths out the emotions, especially anger and grief, while introducing the element of play, two qualities important in the promotion of peace. This essential oil opens and moves energy that is bound up due to fears of retaliation, persecution and dominance. It softens rigidity and the lack of flexibility and encourages imagination and the blissful freedom of play. It utilizes play and laughter to dissolve the pains of betrayal. It allows in truth, in a direct way, through humor. Blue Tansy is a systemic nervous relaxant, analgesic and anti-inflammatory. The essential oil is effective in treating hypertonic conditions, pain management and the healing of wounds.

Blue Tansy

Green Myrtle (*Myrtle communis*) - The ancient Persians regarded myrtle as a holy plant. Myrtle was a symbol of love and peace to the Jews and Greeks and was regarded as sacred. This peaceful heritage is why green myrtle is used here. It is described as a gentle oil which is regenerating, astringent and anti-allergenic. Myrtle essential oil has clarifying, cleansing, refreshing and uplifting properties. It's clarifying properties helps to support decision making and the execution of plans. It is an oil that is emotionally cleansing, curbing self-defeating feelings and addictions. It creates balance and encourages expression, promoting motivation, self confidence and self esteem. Myrtle helps to bring things to the conscious mind.

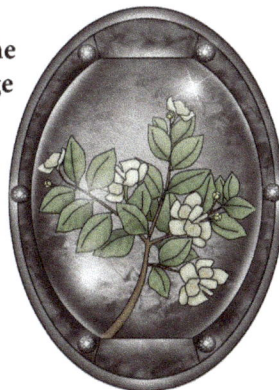

49

Green Myrtle

"Peace"

Essences and Their Functions

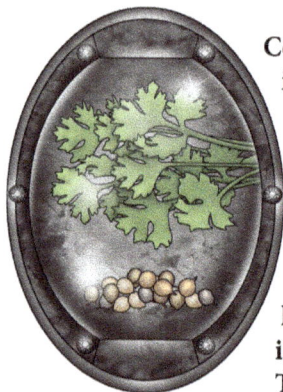

Coriander Seed

Coriander Seed (*Coriandrum sativum*) - Coriander, the herb, is used in many of our kitchens and is recognized as food. As such, coriander seed essential oil is used here to nourish and fill our mind-body. Physically, it helps digestion and transforms dampness. Emotionally, this essential oil fills the spaces of lack or less than. This includes feelings of abandonment, insecurity and bitterness, which may constrict the throat. Here coriander seed helps us find our voice and speak our truth. It can also alleviate feelings of hopelessness, worry, shock and fear, as we feel supported from the inside, from our own power... trusting in our own bodies to heal. This oil originates from Poland.

Saro (*Cinnamosma fragrans*) is an understudied but engaging plant from Madagascar. The essential oil is obtained by steam distillation of the fresh leaves. It has a camphoraceous fragrance profile with smooth, warm, sweet and slightly spicy middle notes that is uplifting and vitalizing, as well as decongesting. Generally, it is used to support immunity, but in this blend it's primarily used for its emotional and spiritual properties. Saro opens and reconnects us to ourselves, to others and to universal energies. It imparts a dignified, connected presence. This essential oil encourages a shift from a disconnected ego based power to a true power that is connected to source. It allows one to live from a trusting, integrated space.

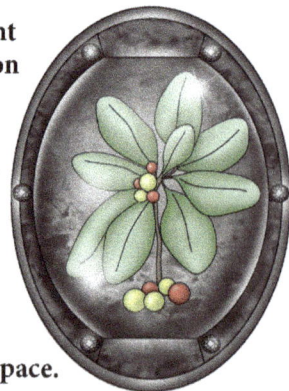

Saro

"Peace"

Peace is the fifth and last protocol of Soldiers Stories Unwound. As previously stated, these protocols are designed to be progressive in nature, as are the take home remedies. This remedy helps the veteran to feel supported at home, whether or not he or she returns for more treatment. Because this is a progressive series, it is not recommended to revisit any of the previous take home remedies or protocols at this stage. On the other hand, this take home remedy can be recommended for as long as the patient requires. It helps the veteran to embrace a life of independence with confidence and joy while encouraging one to connect and be an integral part of one's community. Progressing to this fifth protocol, Peace is like earning your stripes or a diploma, it signifies achievement to the next level.

Home Remedies

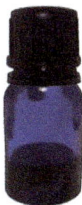

1. Direct inhalation - hold 10 ml bottle of Peace Elixir under nose and take a deep inhale from each nostril. Inhale as needed to feel at peace.

2. Indirect inhalation - drip 5 to 10 drops of Peace Elixir on a tissue upon retiring. Surround nose with tissue and inhale deeply. Slip tissue under the pillow case as you sleep.

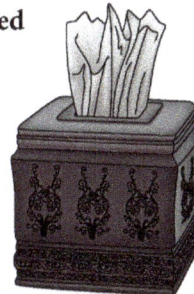

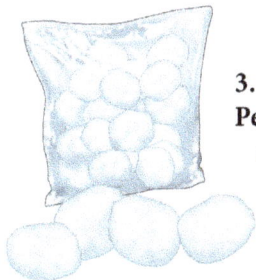

3. Topical application - Upon awakening and after washing, apply Peace Elixir using the snowflake technique, to lower back and abdomen (CV4/GV4). Rest for 10 minutes before starting your day. Use entire bottle using any or all of these three methods.

Essential Oil Application Techniques

Direct Application

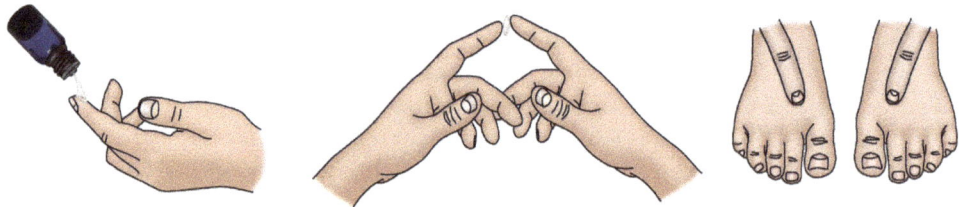

Apply 1-2 drops of elixir on index finger. Transfer elixir to index finger on the opposite hand by lightly pressing fingers together. Gently place elixir on acupuncture points bilaterally. (Use just one finger if point is on the midline). Gently hold fingers on the points for at least 1 minute until shift occurs. This can be a deep breath, a sigh, or a relaxation of the body. You may also feel a shift in your own body or consciousness. Treat this as a mindful or sacred moment.

Indirect Applications

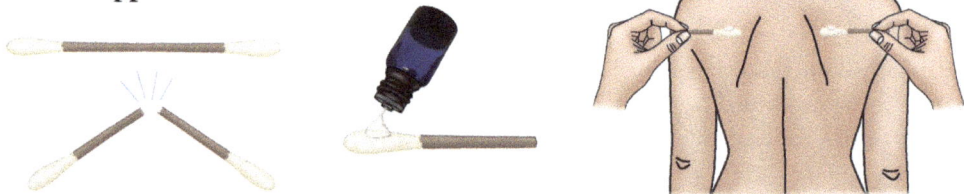

Take a cotton tipped stick, such as a Q-tip, and break or cut in half. Apply 1-2 drops of elixir on both cotton tips. Lightly place on acupuncture points bilaterally or just use one cotton tip if treating a point on the midline. Gently hold for at least 1 minute as described in direct application above. This technique can also be used in the Raindrop Application to follow.

Essential Oil Application Techniques

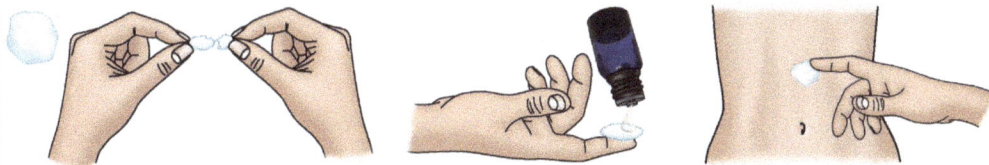

Tear one or two thin pieces of cotton from a cotton ball until it has an appearance of a snow-flake or galaxy. Apply 1-2 drops of elixir on the thin pieces of cotton and transfer them bilaterally onto the acupuncture points being treated. (Use one piece of cotton if the point treated is on the midline). Gently hold with finger for 1 minute until shift occurs as previously described in Direct Application. Cotton will keep essential oils from evaporating quickly.

Raindrop Application

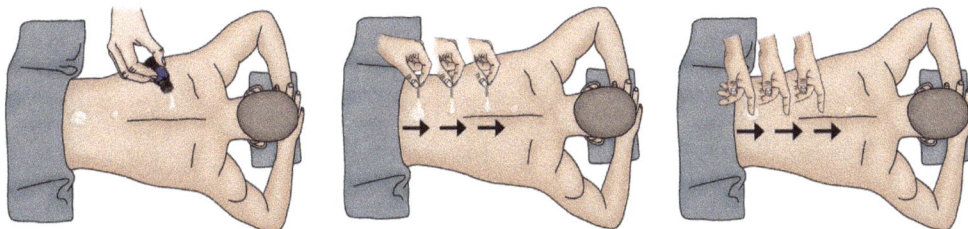

This application can be distributed by direct or indirect methods. Create a small pool of elixir at the base of spine by dripping 5-6 drops on the small of the back . Then drip 1 drop of elixir up the spine every 3 inches. Continue the raindrops along additional pathways as treatment requires. Using cotton tipped sticks or the index and middle fingers of one hand, slowly make a circle in the pool of elixir at the base of spine for 2 or 3 turns and slowly continue connecting the drops of elixir up the spine and through other pathways. Repeat tracing pathway for 2 or 3 more passes. The key is to move as slowly and mindfully as possible.

General References

Craydon, Deborah. *Flora Corona, Hawaiian Flower Essence & Gem Elixir Repertory.* www.floracorona.com, 2012

Gian, Marc. *Holistic Aromatherapy, Practical Self-Healing with Essential Oils.* Cico Books, 2017

Hall, Judy. *The Crystal Bible, A Definitive Guide to Crystals.* Walking Stick Press, 2019

Holmes, Peter. *Aromatica, a Clinical Guide to Essential Oil Therapeutics.* Singing Dragon, 2016

Pollard, Tiffany. *Healing Oil Collective.* master-healer.teachable.com, 2018

Pollard, Tiffany. *Master Healer handouts*, 2015

Shute, Judith. *Foundations of Aromatherapy Certification Program,* aromatic studies.com, 2020

Tisserand & Young. *Essential Oil Safety.* Churchill Livingstone, 2014

Yin Yang House. theory.yinyanghouse.com. 2020

www.ingramcontent.com/pod-product-compliance
Lightning Source LLC
Chambersburg PA
CBHW051559030426
42334CB00031B/3262